Yoga

The All-in-One Yoga Guide – 70 Poses for Every Skillset

D1311200

Yoga

The All-in-One Yoga Guide – 70 Poses for Every Skillset

By Roberto Zanon

© Copyright 2015 Roberto Zanon

This document is geared towards providing exact and reliable information in regards to the topic and issue covered. The publication is sold with the idea that the publisher is not required to render accounting, officially permitted, or otherwise, qualified services. If advice is necessary, legal or professional, a practiced individual in the profession should be ordered.

- From a Declaration of Principles which was accepted and approved equally by a Committee of the American Bar Association and a Committee of Publishers and Associations.

Table of Contents

Getting Started

The word 'Yoga' derives from the word 'yuj' in Sanskrit, meaning 'to unite.' This is appropriate given the multitude of purposes that yoga serves. Aside from the core reality that like-minded people from around the world come together quite often to share in its experience, yoga itself represents the unity of many different principles that can serve our everyday needs.

If you're reading this book you've already taken a step in the right direction. Yoga not only helps the practitioner get into better physical shape, it's a holistically beneficial activity. This book is going to help you approach yoga as a beginner and give you some tips to succeed in your quest for a better mind, spirit and body, which is what the practice of yoga is all about. Yoga's benefits are innumerable.

It's important to first dispel some of the myths about yoga. Despite being an activity that is sometimes associated with the feminine, there are many males that participate in the practice and there are a high number of male teachers. Some types of yoga, such as Hatha Flow, the most popular, are quite strenuous; enough so that it should instantly debunk any myths about yoga is too girly an activity for blustery males. Some also tend to believe that you need to be flexible to do yoga. This is patently untrue. Many yogis are not flexible at all, though the practice encourages them to expand their flexibility over time. Part of the rationale of yoga is accepting that bodies are unique and different. Respecting the limitations of your body is key and is also important in avoiding injury.

First let's discuss the body. Yoga has rejuvenating effects that surprise even veterans. A standard class lasts one and a half hours, and classes are often very strenuous. Yet at the end of them, yogis do not feel emptied of energy but just the opposite. Rather, they quite often feel energetic and ready for their day. Yoga classes are typically held throughout the day, running from as early as 5am to 7pm at night. Exercises are also extremely balanced, meaning that they practically focus on the body as a whole, rather than just one small part. In this book, students of yoga are referred to as 'yogis.' Experienced employees leading the class are simply called 'teachers' or 'yoga teachers.'

Avoiding Injury

Yoga is a very safe activity, as the entire practice typically takes place on a solitary mat. I can't really stress enough the importance of a Yoga mat as new students sometimes overlook this. A very economic, yet high quality Yoga mat I have already found is this one. However an in any physical endeavor, especially involving strenuous exercise, there is a risk of overdoing things and injuring yourself. Here are a few ways not to do that. First, yoga should generally be avoided by women in the late stages of pregnancy. Generally at this point many of the poses are difficult to begin with. Also if there are prior injuries it's possible to exacerbate them. Yoga places a lot of pressure on the feet and the wrists. It isolates different parts of the body generally, and focuses on them one by one. Yogis with prior injuries in these areas could make things worse. Generally in the beginning of the class instructors will ask their students if they have prior injuries. It's important to be honest with them. If you ever need to take a break, particularly if in the course of the practice you are putting pressure on an area that makes you physically uncomfortable, there is nothing wrong with taking a break and going into the child's pose. You can wait there until the focus shifts to another body part. Some of the more challenging poses can be worrisome if the yogi does not have control. Beginners should be careful for instance when they try head stands and shoulder stands in the first few months of their practice. Generally a spotter is required to prevent balance from being lost, which could end up causing a cascade of teetering yogis, knocking each other over like dominos across the room.

Yoga etiquette

It's important to maintain yoga etiquette if you're going to a public class. It's not as if you'll be inundated by tons of different rules, but there are a few basic expectations that it's important to be aware of. The first of these is that you generally want to be early to class, so you have time to set up your mat (or a borrowed one) and get into a relaxed state. Class members sometimes chat when they first arrive, but as it becomes time to begin they are generally expected to fall silent and become attentive to the instructor. Bathroom breaks are fine, but are not all that common. The sessions are rather long (1.5 hours) so it's permissible to leave, but if you do just make sure not to disrupt the class. Some yoga centers may ask that males not take their shirts off during practice or that yogis avoid showing up already emanating unpleasant odors. This may seem strange given that yoga is a highly physical activity, but it's also meant to appeal to the other senses, including smell. There is generally incense burning in the room, so as to make for a pleasant aroma.

The Origin of Yoga

While yoga is a modern activity, it is in fact an ancient practice that has been developing for many centuries in tandem with Hinduism. It celebrates some of the main Hindu beliefs, including those of peace, serenity and harmony with both mankind and nature, the destruction of the ego and a mental flow state that encourages creativity, positivity and originality. Adherence to discipline is also a key belief, as yogis are encouraged to endure the physical and mental hardship of practice for the duration of the class as best they can.

Yoga originates from the Indus civilization, which encompassed 300,000 square miles in part of what is now modern India. Sources differ on the precise date that the practice of yoga began, as this goes back so long that it's difficult to say. There is proof however that yoga has been in practice for at least 5,000 years, based upon depictions of figures in yogic poses in the cities of Daro, Harappa and Mohenjo found by archaeologists. Yet there are indications that yoga may have been in existence for possibly even up to 17,000 years. This has led to a deep, wise and streamlined practice that has stood the test of time.

Just because the practice has been around for so long doesn't necessarily mean that it has always existed in the form that it's in today. It has gone through many different permutations throughout its long journey before it became popular in western civilization. In fact, Hatha, which is perhaps the most pervasive form of yoga today, was created in the 4th and 5th centuries, and took centuries to become culturally relevant around the world. Many practitioners and gurus (or teachers) who have decided to make yoga a top priority in their lives have gone to India to practice, where yoga is taught in a manner that is considered the closest to its purest form possible.

Teacher training is popular in India as well and often linked closely to lengthy sessions of vows of silence and meditation. Travelers have found India to be a spectacular destination; though it is one with which many yogis have a love/hate relationship. It is both one of the most beautiful travel destinations in the world and one of the most challenging, especially during attempts to explore the 'real India', outside the comfort of tourist zones and luxury. Learning more about the origin of yoga will enrich your experience, and put you in touch with the fundamental principles, which can be life changing additions to its physical benefits.

The Standard Format

This chapter discusses the many different forms of yoga to help guide the reader in deciding where to start, and eventually how to manage his or her time when it comes to your personal practice. It should be noted that although most yoga centers also sometimes offer alternative classes like Salsa and Pilates. This is simply because yogis are often interested in these activities as well, and some yoga teachers have skills in both.

While differing in terms of difficulty and style most yoga classes have a similar format. Generally students begin seated on their mats facing the front of the room with their legs crossed. In yoga etiquette all participants usually fall silent and place their attention on the instructor. Talking during the practice is usually limited, although from time to time the instructor will ask whether the students have questions. If there's an emergency of course it's fine to bring an interruption. Aside from this talking during the session on the part of the participants should be generally kept to a minimum. Hands rest on the knees with palms facing upward. Some yogis extend their fingers or put them in a ring configuration, while others just rest them there. Instructors will sometimes come around the room and help the participants by adjusting their posture. Some instructors make a point of asking yogis who are uncomfortable being touched to signify this somehow, usually by turning one corner of their mat under. If you prefer this boundary, this is an option.

The teacher will also ask the participants to sit up as straight as possible and tilt their heads slightly back. At first this can be difficult, particularly for participants who are accustomed to slouching. Over time however one becomes accustomed to this pose, and it makes a giant improvement to posture, which helps maintain the health of the back over the long term. Different teachers have different styles. Some prefer to give speeches at the beginning of the session. These often adhere to different themes, like positivity, discipline or perseverance and are designed to share some of the ancient spoken wisdom that comes from the practice of yoga. Other teachers prefer not to talk much in the beginning and get right into the practice. Before the physical activity begins there is a session of ohms, when participants are asked to mimic the teacher's sounds vocally. This tends to put the class in sync. Generally this is short as well. If you don't feel comfortable participating verbally you aren't required to do so, but in order to get the full experience of the session participants are usually encouraged to trust the leadership of the instructor.

Classes typically start with easier stretches that are integrated into the program. Stretching in the beginning is not like stretching before a sports practice. It's part of the fabric of yoga itself. This may seem strange but if participants simply follow the instruction of the teacher it is made easy. Instructors often mimic the poses that they ask their students to do to give examples. If a student is having difficulty getting into a pose, an instructor will generally step over and help guide him or her. This is quite common too with handstands and headstands, which are some of the more difficult and precarious positions in yoga. When a yogi is guided by a spotter they become much easier. Then over time students can learn to do these poses on their own.

Although not always performing strenuous activity throughout the entirety of the practice, participants are always kept more or less 'busy' or occupied. There are no real breaks but there are periodic resting times where the child's pose is used, most often just after the most strenuous portions of the practice. Usually in the beginning the pace is slow, and it often begins to speed up significantly about twenty minutes into the practice. Some poses focus on the legs (or one leg at a time) while others focus on the upper body. Often there are variations of a pose based upon relative difficulty, and these are described by the instructor to allow the students to choose the pose that suits them best.

Periodic breaks are given throughout. Near the end of the practice instructors resort to 'cool down' poses which are intended to bring the body back into a state of rest and relaxation. Practice ends with the savasana, in which the students lie on their backs, usually for about five to ten minutes to the sound of soothing music or silence. This is a kind of meditation period in which chants or relaxing words are spoken by the instructor. After the savasana, students sit up again as in the beginning of the practice session with their legs crossed, arms resting on their knees, and palms open upward. Chants are repeated again.

Showing Up

It may be a little intimidating showing up to your first yoga class, so this chapter fleshes out what the experience is like to show fresh yogis that yoga studios are casual environments. Remember also that you're there to maintain a state of low stress. You want to get a workout in and possibly to engage in meditation. Anxiety is the last thing you should want to experience. If you're feeling out of shape, don't compare your body to others'. Yoga is supposed to be all about self-improvement, and while some yogis are particularly proud of their achievements, communities are generally very welcoming. That said there seldom needs to be any conversing involved before class begins. Plenty of yogis prefer to set up their mats silently without talking to anyone, as a way to prepare themselves mentally for practice.

The teacher may ask the yogis to raise their hands if it is their first class. This happens more often in difficult classes, where there can be concern that a beginner has mistakenly wandered into a class too advanced for him or her. Despite its reputation as a primarily feminine activity, yoga can be an incredibly strenuous activity, pushing the limits of one's physical cardio, balance and longevity.

Before you go, check the schedule to see if the classes are numbered in terms of difficulty. It's recommended that beginners start out with at least one 'intro' class. That way they can broadly and slowly introduce themselves to the different core poses without feeling the pressure of quick transitions, which are often quite difficult even for very experienced yogis.

Beginners should always remember that if they get too tired to keep up with the rest of the class during session, it's perfectly fine to return to the 'child's position', which is designed for rest. Teachers should introduce this early-on to beginners. The chin is tucked in while the knees are bent and tucked into the chest. Toes are pointed while the body leans forward on the legs. This pose is not always comfortable at first, but becomes comfortable with time.

Some beginners are worried about needing equipment for yoga, but this is not the case. That's one of the beauties of this practice. All you need to do is show up wearing workout gear. For ladies a pushup bra and yoga pants are fine, but gym shorts work just as well. Some yogis make a point of their yoga fashion getup. If that's part of a ritual that adds meaning to the practice for you, then it's certainly worth it. But having special yoga pants isn't going to give you a better workout. What's more important is your attentiveness and adherence to the teacher's direction, your breathing and self-awareness, your developing agility and balance, and your self-improvement over time. For those that really care about the core significance of yoga, fashion is a superficial element. It is sometimes helpful to remember that Lululemon didn't exist thousands of years ago in India where yoga was developed, when fashion in yoga was less of a priority. Don't scrutinize your clothes as much as you do your technique and commitment. This doesn't mean that yogis should feel bad if they can't go every day, but focus in the moment is a key priority.

As for mats, they are made available for use already, so you can just borrow them at the studio. You don't need any other equipment. Just bring your body and a positive attitude. Aside from that, you're ready to go! Happy practice!

Popular Types of Yoga

The following forms of yoga are some of the most popular. Take a look below to see what you think might fit you best in getting started out. Naturally over the long term it is healthy to expand your horizons and try new forms of yoga as much as possible. You never know. It could become your favorite new thing! Descriptions include difficulty levels along with the general focus of the class.

Hatha (Flow)

Hatha focuses on body movements designed to break a sweat through compound exercises that divide the body into quarters. Generally it has a heavy focus on building leg strength and leg balance at the same time, transitioning then into an upper-body focus, which includes push-up like motions in short repetition. Ordinary hatha classes focus on holding one or more positions for longer periods of time whereas hatha flow classes feature more rapid movement for the purpose of getting a more active workout.

Vinyasa (Flow)

Vinyasa classes are a form of Hatha yoga designed to focus on the more physical aspect of yogic exercise within the standard format of a yoga class, including chants in the beginning and a savasana at the end. The core format is for participants to periodically come to rest in the downward dog position, sometimes transitioning back to plank, then leaping with the feet forward such that they're positioned next to the hands. The next step is to reach the hands high up in the air, then down again to the feet, leap backwards, then drop the body down in a push-up fashion to the ground yet without making full contact with the chest. Pushing the body up again as the legs are straight and the feet are pointing backwards, the body transitions into downward dog and then plank position. This process begins slow and gradually increases in speed. Other stretches and exercises are integrated, but generally this routine is what gives the practice its continuity.

Meditation

While many classes are quite physically active, others focus almost entirely on meditation and on linking meditation to breathing exercises. Those who do not meditate on a regular basis will want to start with a lower level class, as the higher level classes often require that participants meditate for longer periods of time. Generally, the meditation sessions in beginner level classes last for around fifteen minutes with some occasional physical exercises to stretch out the body and create some contrast during the class. Meditation focuses on relaxing the body completely and exiting all thoughts from the mind, striving to attain a new height of focus and consciousness.

Teachers often guide participants through different mantras that help one to attain this state of mind.

Readers should remember that there are many different kinds of meditation as well. Some focus particularly on the release of physical and emotional pain, involving a chance for venting. Students are generally encouraged not just to meditate during class, but at home as well. 10 minutes of meditation every day can make a huge difference, and change one's perspective on life.

Breathing Classes

Breathing classes are often held in yoga centers. These include a variety of different techniques, which try to heighten consciousness through rapid breathing, circular breathing, and the syncopation of breathing with different physical exercises. Breathing exercises border on a kind of hyperventilation, which can be exhilarating, and rehabilitating with respect to the mind and consciousness. The beauty of these exercises is that once learned they can be done nearly anywhere.

Pilates

Although not technically yoga, and developed much more recently, pilates exercises share many of the same movements and concepts as yoga, with a focus on developing the muscles in the core, enhancing balance, breathing, and centering exercises. The concept of centering derives from understanding the core as being the center of intent and identity aside from just the development of the abdominal muscles. Pilates is more an exercise-centric activity than yoga, which embodies a more spiritual aspect.

Nutrition and Yoga

As I mentioned earlier, it wasn't just yoga poses that helped me lose weight. I had to change my eating habits, too. You see, as we age, our bodies need less carbohydrates to keep them fueled because we're not running around like we were when we were seven or eight. Yet most of us don't change our eating habits that much throughout our lives and we end up with a lot of extra fuel in our body that's converted into fat.

When I realized I wanted to lose weight and be fit, I immediately started doing the research on how our bodies store fat. What I found is there's a lot of contradictory information out there. In short, scientists don't know everything about our bodies thus far, but they do know a few things.

This is what I found:

There are several steps for proteins to turn into fat. First, you ingest some type of food with protein such as meat or fish. Let me clarify, we're talking about animal proteins and not vegetable proteins, which are processed differently. Once the meat is broken down into the protein, it's then turned into an amino acid. From there, it travels to the liver and is converted into glucose. Glucose must bind with insulin in order to create a fatty acid. That fatty acid is then used as fuel, and if there's too many left over, then the body stores it as fat.

Nuts and seeds that are mainly fat already are broken down into their fat molecules and converted directly into fatty acids. So as you can see, nuts and seeds take a lot less time and energy to be broken down into body fat.

All other carbohydrates such as starchy vegetables, grains, and fruits are converted to glucose, which is then bound with insulin to form a fatty acid. This is also a rather quick process.

Digesting proteins takes a lot longer and a lot more energy, which means that if we're only ingesting high amounts of protein and vegetables that are non-starchy, we'll be expending energy to digest the food and it'll be easier for us to lose weight. So long story short, I switched my diet to one with higher amounts of protein, fiber, and non-starchy vegetables. I had to cut out the candies, cookies, and other carbohydrate rich foods for a while, but now I can eat them in moderation and not worry about gaining weight.

It's all about finding your limits and knowing them. So let's move on from diet and get right into the poses!

Core Positions and Progression

You'll learn these if you take a beginner's class, but just to familiarize the reader with them, here are some of the core positions in yoga. These are generally the first things that a beginner learns when he or she comes to class. It's important to do these with correct technique. Otherwise, not only can this be harmful to parts of your body, but your muscle memory could develop the wrong habits, which is not the best path for advancement!

Now that you have a lot of the basics about yoga you'll be at an advantage when showing up to your first class. Let's talk a little bit about the process of progressing in yoga. Everyone tends to do so at their own pace, which depends not just on yoga but on consistently making healthy lifestyle choices, as in those that are conducive to your growth physically, mentally and spiritually. The great thing about yoga is that it puts you around people that tend to value healthy lifestyles. Their food choices and habits are likely to influence your own, and thus will result in even greater benefits over the long run.

There's an old saying that if you want to learn something fast, learn it slow, and if you want to learn it slow, learn it fast. Yoga is not a thing to be rushed, although when you do practice, it deserves your full attention and commitment. Those who periodically take breaks from yoga may also find that their time off has allowed them to process some of the body movements, and are surprised at how easy it is to return. If you simply commit to doing your best and go on a regular basis you will improve, and you're certain to see the results.

*Note: I have marked every Yoga pose with an indicative difficulty level system – 1 star being the easiest ones, to 5 stars for the most advanced ones - in case you want to escalate from the most basic ones to the most advanced.

Downward Dog (★☆☆☆☆)

In this position the yogi is facing downward (true to its name), supported by both hands and feet in what should look essentially like an upside down 'V'. The back should be straight while the arms are outstretched forward and parallel to each other. Harm can come to the wrists by being in this position while the wrists are rotated inward or outward. Yogis should try to move their feet closer to their hands. Some try to flatten their feet, though this is not possible for some. At first this is a difficult pose to hold for long periods of time. However later on it becomes a comfortable spot for resting.

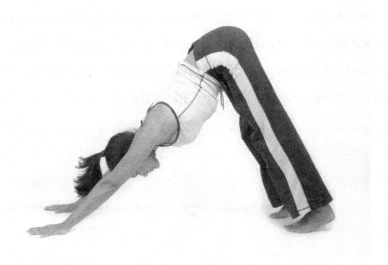

Warrior Pose (1, 2 & 3) (★☆☆☆☆)

The warrior pose begins with one leg extended out in front of the body, foot flat on the floor and knee at a right angle, while the other leg is extended backwards and remains straight. The back leg is supported by standing on the toes. Meanwhile the arms are outstretched in the direction consistent with legs i.e. right leg forward, right arm forward, left leg backward, left arm backward. This describes the warrior pose 1. Usually afterward this transitions into warrior pose 2, in which the only thing that changes is that the hands move to being outstretched at the sides. In warrior pose 3 the back foot is lifted up into the air such that the balance is kept on only the front foot while both arms remain outstretched to the sides. This works out the solo leg in addition to being a challenging balance exercise. Moving through these phases with finesse and control is also part of the challenge, as is letting the airborne foot down gradually and softly.

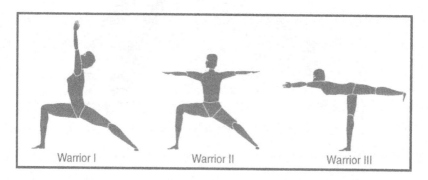

Warrior I   Warrior II   Warrior III

Cat-Cow Stretch (★☆☆☆☆)

This begins on the hands and knees, head facing upward and back facing straight. It transitions to the head facing down and the back arching. This is considered a way of opening up the heart and loosening up the mid-section. This is also a core position from which the legs can be extended one by one, testing endurance. A more advanced variation involves lifting the hand on the opposite side of your body and outstretching it forward or straight to the side. This manifests a challenge for balance as well.

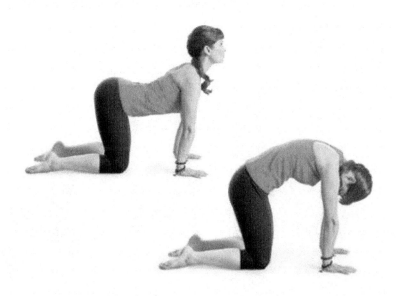

Child's Pose (★☆☆☆☆)

Child's pose is excellent for stretching out your lower back and realigning your discs, as well as stretching and strengthening your hips. This pose is used to relieve stress, abdominal upset, fatigue, and lower back discomfort. If you're someone who sits in a chair all day at work, then you would benefit from Child's Pose. To perform the pose, you would sit on your heels with your hands on your thighs and lower your chest to the rest on your thighs. Bring your forehead down to the floor and relax your arms beside your legs with your palms facing the ceiling. Hold this pose for five to ten deep breaths and then slowly sit up. If you still feel tight in your back or you're still stressed, try to meditate while in this pose.

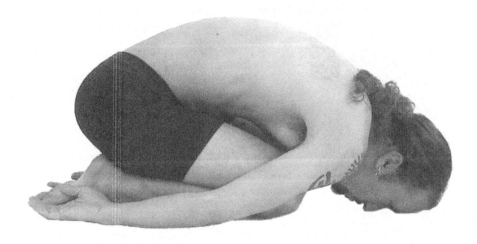

Child's Pose, Wide-Kneed Variation (★☆☆☆☆)

Sometimes you need to perform a pose that's a little more widening to help you stretch your lower and upper back muscles, as well as your hips, thighs, and groin area. If you're experiencing indigestion or a scattered mind, the wide-kneed variation of child's pose is an excellent one to start with. Simply get into position for downward-facing dog. Now lift your heels and separate your knees while you lower down to the floor. Lower your body to the mat and keep your hands stretched in front of you instead of beside you. Your knees should be a little bit apart and your arms stretched out straight.

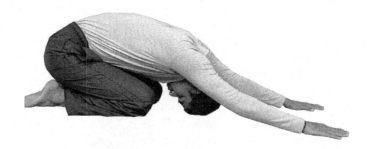

Knees to Chest (★☆☆☆☆)

The knees to chest position is excellent for beginners and helps relieve digestive upset as well as relieve stress. If you have a tight back, then you should do this pose. To perform the pose, lie down on your back and put your feet flat on the floor with your knees bent. Your arms should be stretched out beside your body with your palms facing up. Bring your knees to your chest and place your right hand on your right shin as well as your left hand on your left shin. Pull you knees toward you. Wrap your arms around your legs until the inside of your elbows are touching your legs, and then grasp hold of your right elbow with your left hand and your left elbow with your right hand. Rock back and forth ten times gently and then release your elbows. Keep your right hand on your right knee and your left hand on your left knee, and make ten circles with your legs and hips. Keep the legs together.

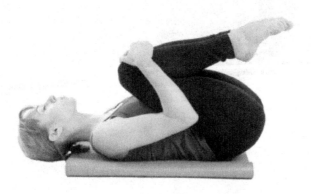

Legs Up The Wall (★★☆☆☆)

If you have tight hamstrings, chest, abs, and neck muscles, then the legs up the wall position will be good for you. People who suffer from tired legs and feet, anxiety, insomnia, stress, and a scattered mind should perform this position. To do the position, start by sitting with your knees bent and the left side of your body up against the wall. Place your palms on the floor beside your hips and turn your hips so that they're facing the wall while you swing your legs up. Your head should be back and your legs should be touching the wall. Place your buttocks against the wall so that you're straight. Hold for five to ten deep breaths.

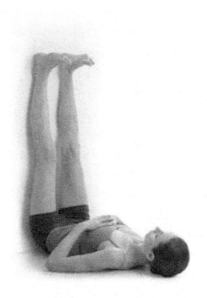

Mountain Pose (★☆☆☆☆)

The mountain pose has to be one of the easiest physical poses out there in yoga, but you have to have a focused mind while you do it. It's for strengthening your back, legs, abs, and spine. People who have poor posture and a scattered mind should try this pose. Simply stand with your feet together and your big toes touching. You should be looking forward and not down. Now, tighten your thigh muscles, active your kneecaps, broaden your collarbone and stretch your arms down alongside your body. Hold for five to ten deep breaths.

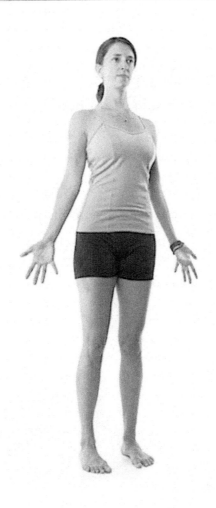

Reclining Twist (★★☆☆☆)

The reclining twist is also great for stretching your back, thighs, neck, glutes, and spine. Lie down on your back and extend your arms out straight from your shoulders. Shift your hips to the right and cross your right thigh over your left thigh. Now lift your legs up into the air and pull your knees a little closer to your torso. Allow your legs to drop to the left as you look the right. Hold for five to ten breaths and then switch sides.

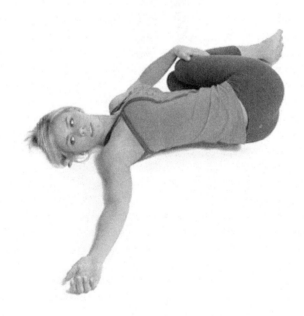

Seated Forward Bend (★★☆☆☆)

While it looks pretty easy, the seated forward bend is a little more difficult to perform if you're not very flexible. This is for stretching out your back, legs, and lengthening your spine. If you suffer from digestive upset and headaches, try this move. Sit in staff position with your legs out in front of you, your ankles touching, and your back and spine straight. Now inhale and place your arms above your head at shoulder width apart. Exhale and reach your arms forward until you can grasp hold of our toes, shins, or knees. Go only as far as you are comfortable. Lower your head between your shoulders or touch your forehead to your knees if you can. Hold this position for five breaths and then slowly sit up.

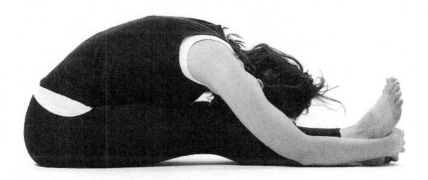

Seated Twist (★★☆☆☆)

The seated twist will stretch your hips and help with constipation or diarrhea. To perform this pose, sit in the agnistambhasana pose with your right foot on your left knee and your left foot on your right knee. Move your right leg with your hands and put the sole of your right foot on the floor next to your left knee. Your right toes should be facing forward. Now move your left foot back and bring the left heel next to your right hip. Extend your left arm up as you inhale, bend it and put your elbow and upper arm on the right side of your right knee. Put your right hand behind you. Place your left elbow into your right knee and twist your torso until your facing to the side. Put your left hand on the outside of your right hip to hold your position.

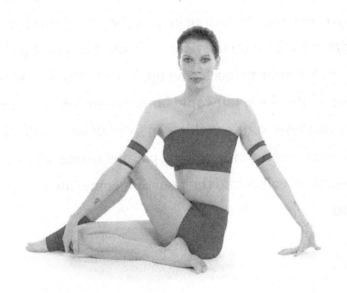

Sphinx Pose (★★☆☆☆)

The sphinx pose is great for stretching out your chest and your back. If you experience back pain, you should try this pose. Lie down with your front on the floor and your arms alongside your body with your palms facing up. Your forehead and toes should be on the floor. Lift your shoulders and chest and put your elbows under your shoulders in front of you on the floor. Let your forearms rest on the floor parallel to one another. Now press your palms into the floor and come into a slight backbend.

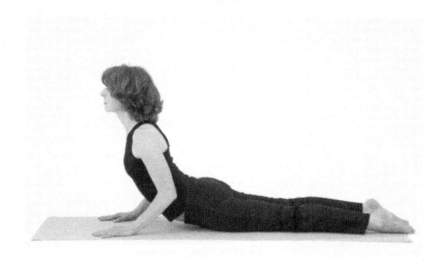

Squat Pose (★★☆☆☆)

Warning: You should not perform this pose if you are pregnant. Otherwise, the squat pose is excellent for strengthening your back, hips, thighs, and buttocks. To perform this pose, stand with your feet parallel and hip width apart. Turn your toes out at a forty-five degree angle and then bend your knees and lower your butt into a squat. Your torso should be upright and our palms together at your chest. Press your elbows outward against the inside of your knees and hold for five to ten breaths.

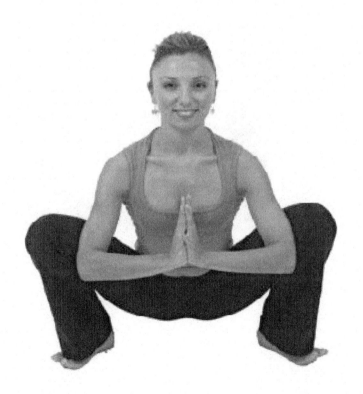

Staff Pose (★☆☆☆☆)

Excellent for strengthening your thighs, core, and back, the staff pose is very easy to perform. Simply sit with your legs out in front of you and your ankles touching. Your toes should be pointing up. Place your hands next to your hips and slide your shoulder blades downward. Broaden your chest and reach forward through the inner edges of your feet and look straight ahead. Hold for five to ten deep breaths.

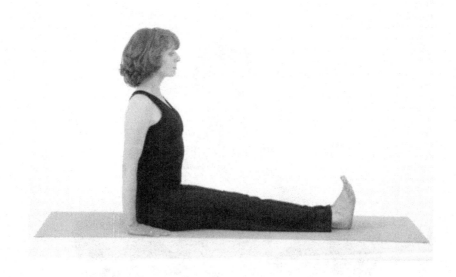

Standing Forward Bend (★★★☆☆)

This might be considered one of the harder beginner moves because while it looks easy, it requires balance and flexibility. Start by standing in the mountain pose and bring your hands to a prayer position in front of you, palms together. Inhale and gaze up at the ceiling, lifting your chest as you do so. Then exhale and fold forward starting at the hips and keeping your spine straight. Do not allow your hips to get behind your ankles! Now bring your palms to the floor if you can, or fingertips, or grasp your shins if you must. Inhale and exhale five times, and then come back to the mountain pose.

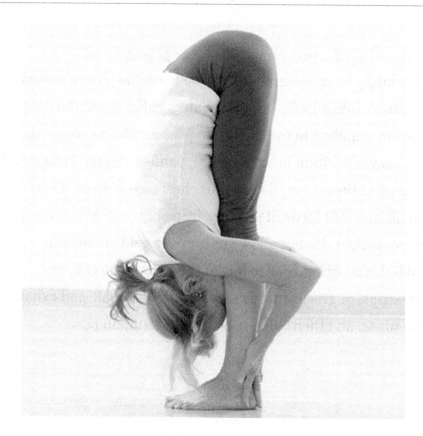

Savasana (★☆☆☆☆)

The Savasana is the final pose in yoga, done at the end of every yoga practice. It is part resting, part meditation and part focusing on your purpose for the practice and on the effect you intend for it to have on your life. Though this is the least difficult pose of all physically, it has been said that there is no pose more difficult than the Savasana, because penetrating the core of its meaning involves a state of consciousness that requires unique experience and focus.

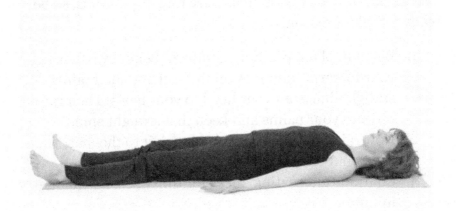

Cha-Cha (★☆☆☆☆)

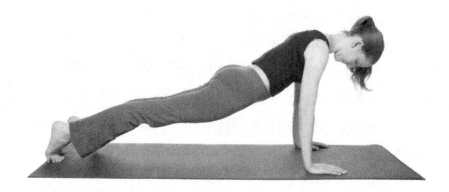

Photo courtesy of dgilder at Flickr.com

It sounds fun, and it is fun! Especially if you're motivated to lose weight *and* look good. This pose targets your abs, so be ready for bikini season!

1. Begin in plank position as shown. Begin by balancing your forearms and toes on the mat and maintain a straight line from your head to your heels. Then raise up onto your palms and keep that straight spine.
2. Now raise your left knee and touch it to the mat. Then right your right knee and touch it to the mat.
3. Continue alternating knees for thirty seconds to one minute.

High Heel (★★☆☆☆)

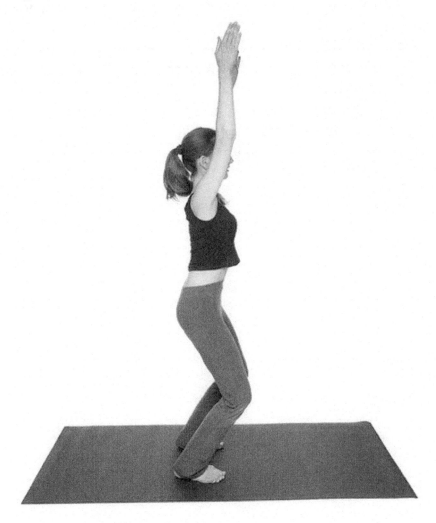

Photo courtesy of dgilder at Flickr.com

It may not sound difficult, but you'll see that it works out your butt, legs, and abs all at once when you try it!

1. Begin in the chair pose like you did for the first exercise. Stand with your feet together and your arms above your head with your palms facing each other. Now sink down into a squat.
2. Pull both your heels off the mat and lower your arms in front of you so that they're at shoulder length. Rise onto your tiptoes.
3. Do three pulses of lowering your butt two inches toward your heels and raising it again.
4. Lower your heels and return to the standing chair position.
5. Do this ten times.

Pendulum Plank (★★☆☆☆)

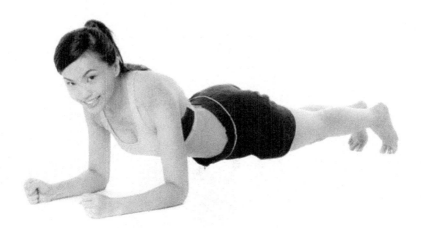

Photo courtesy of Average Moms Wear Capes at Flickr.com

This plank position is a little different from the other plank position, so be sure to remember which one you should be using.

1. Start in the plank position shown above. Balance your forearms and your toes on the mat and keep a straight spine from your head to your heels.
2. Lift your left foot a little off the mat and bring it to a forty-five degree angle to your left side. Hold for one count and then return it back to its original position.
3. Repeat the moves with your right leg to make one repetition.
4. Do ten repetitions.

Kickstand Tap (★★★☆☆)

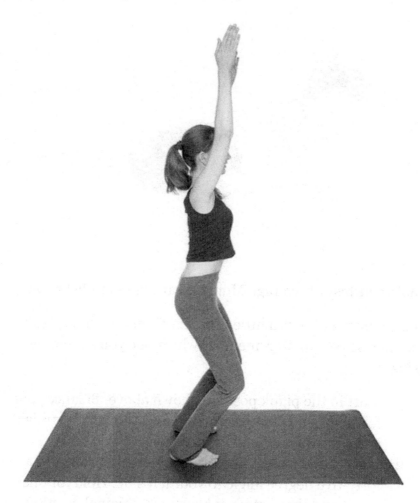

Photo courtesy of dgilder at Flickr.com

The kickstand tap starts out in the chair pose and it's great for tightening your abs, butt and your legs. Be sure to do it slowly the first few times so that you know how you're going to react to moving into these positions, and then kick it up a notch to help with weight loss.

1. Start in the chair pose with your feet together and your arms extended above you with your palms facing each other. Then sink into a squat.
2. Keep squatting, lift your left foot up and put it behind you to tap on the mat. It should be extended as far as you can go comfortably.
3. Bring it back quickly so that you don't lose your balance. Do this twenty times and then switch to your right leg.

If you're having trouble keeping your balance, it might be easier to put your hands on your hips while you're in the squat position.

Side Slide (★★★☆☆)

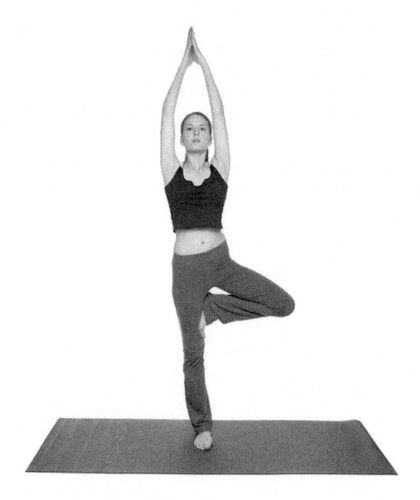

Photo courtesy of dgilder at Flickr.com

The side slide is excellent for strengthening your abs, chest, butt, hips and legs. If you're not good at balancing, you might want to practice that before you do this move.

1. Begin in the tree pose with your palms together in front of your chest and bend your right knee out. Place your

right foot on the inner thigh of your left leg and extend your arms upward, or keep them in front of you. This is a personal choice.

2. Bend your left knee as you lower into a squat and extend your right leg directly to the side. Your toes should be pointing forward and your entire foot should be on the floor.

3. Return to the tree pose and tap your right foot to your inner left thigh and then repeat the move.

4. Do twenty repetitions and then switch to the other side.

Sumo Warrior (★★★☆☆)

I think you're really going to like this one! It combines the warrior pose II, squats, and the heel exercise we did earlier. So it'll shape your butt, quads, calves, abs, and shoulders.

1. Begin in warrior II pose. Stand with your feet in line with your hips and your arms extended out to the sides, your palms should be facing down. Lunge with your left leg out to the left side and point the toes to the left. Now your knee should be over your ankle and your right leg should be straight. Turn your head to the left to following the line of sight of your arm.

2. Pivot your heels so that your toes are turned slightly outward and look forward. Now sink into a squat.

3. Lift your heels off the mat and do three pulses, lowering your butt two inches toward your heels and rising back into the squat.

4. Pivot your feet so that you're returned to warrior II pose and then face right. Point your right toes to the right and your left toes forward. Lean your body weight over your bent, right leg and straighten your left leg as you look to the right. This is one rep.

5. Do six repetitions.

Running Dog (★★★☆☆)

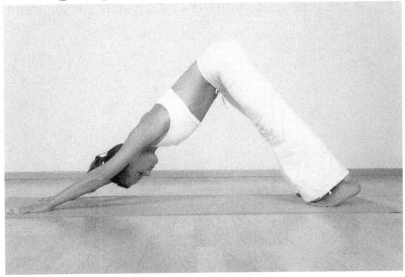

Photo courtesy of wldplan at Flickr.com

Running dog is pretty interesting, to say the least. It will strengthen your arms, butt, core, and your hamstrings, so pretty much your entire body.

1. Begin in downward dog as pictured above. Get down on all fours on the mat with your knees on the floor and your hands on the floor, pointing out. Tuck your toes under you and press your hips back and to the ceiling. Your feet should step back a few inches and you should form an inverted 'V'. Your palms should be flat on the floor and your heels should be touching the floor. If you're heels cannot touch the floor, go only as far as you comfortably can.

2. Keep your 'V' position and bring your left knee in toward your chest. Press the left heel back to extend your leg directly into the air behind you. Bring your

knee in again and then place your foot back on the floor.

3. Do ten repetitions and then switch sides for ten more.

Scorpion Press (★★★☆☆)

The scorpion press starts out in the downward dog position, too, so refer to the previous photograph for instructions. This move will strengthen your butt, legs, core, and arms.

1. Begin in downward dog by kneeling on all fours and then tuck your toes underneath and move your feet a few inches back as you raise your hips to the ceiling. Remember, your palms should be touching the floor and your heels should be touching, but go only as far as you comfortably can.

2. Now, maintain your inverted 'V' position and lift your right foot off the mat. Bend your right knee at ninety degrees and raise your leg so that your right thigh is in line with your back.

3. Keep your bent right leg in the air and then bend your left leg ninety degrees. Lower your knee to the floor and straighten it again.

4. Do ten repetitions and then switch legs.

Hip Shaper (★★★★☆)

Refer to the aforementioned picture for tree pose if you're confused about the instructions for this.

1. Begin in tree pose, standing with your palms together in front of your chest and your left knee out to the side with your left foot on the inner part of your right thigh.
2. Keep your left foot on your right thigh and bring your left knee across your body to the right. And extend your left leg out to the right.
3. Bend your left knee, and bring it out to the left side to return to tree pose.
4. Do ten repetitions and then switch sides to repeat.

Warrior Windmill (★★★★☆)

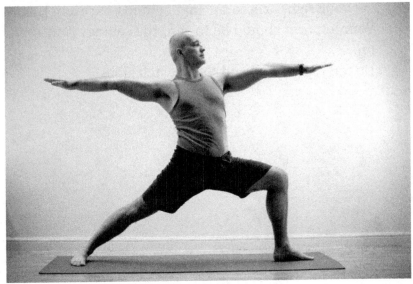

Photo courtesy of Bonar at Flickr.com

The warrior windmill is another one where you're going to need excellent balance, but if you can pull it off, you'll be strengthening your abs, shoulders, butt, oblique, and your legs.

1. Star in the warrior II pose as pictured. You'll need to stand with your feet apart at hips' width and your arms extended out to your sides. Your palms should be facing down. Then lunge with your right leg out to the right and put your toes pointing right. Place your knee over the ankle and your let leg should be straight. Turn your head to the right.
2. Keep this lunge position throughout the exercise.
3. Hinge at your waist to the left and bring your left hand toward the mat by your outside left ankle. Bring your right arm overhead.

4. Keep your feet planted and quickly reverse the direction of your windmill; bring your hinge toward the right and arc your right arm to the mat behind your right thigh. Your left arm should be toward the ceiling. That's one rep.

5. Do ten repetitions and then switch sides.

Sun Salutation (★☆☆☆☆)

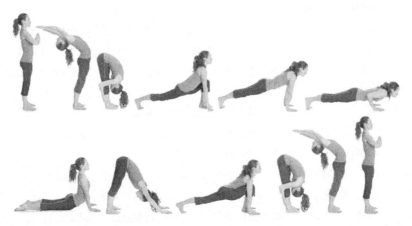

If you really want to get a cardio workout before you begin the aforementioned moves, and as a good way to cool off, do sun salutations. The idea here is to move from one move into the next fluidly.

1. Begin in asana one with your feet hip width apart and your palms in front of you, touching.
2. Now stretch back with your arms straight and your fingers pointing back into asana two.
3. Move into asana three by bending forward and hugging your calves or your thighs if you can't bend too far.
4. Now bring your palms to the floor, step your right leg back and bring your left knee to your chest. This is asana four.
5. In asana five, you'll be moving into plank position. So step your left leg back and bring your palms to the floor as your spine is straightened. Your toes should be touching the floor only.
6. In asana six, you'll be lowering yourself to the floor into the lower position of a push-up, so your upper arms will

be in line with your body or parallel to the floor, and your toes will be touching the floor. You should be looking forward.

7. Bring yourself up into asana seven where your hips are lowered to the ground as you raise your front so that your arms are straight and in line with your body. Keep looking forward.

8. Raise your hips into the air and put your heels flat on the floor along with your palms as you come into downward dog or asana eight.

9. Step your right leg forward and touch your knee to your chest as you bring your body up so that it's parallel with the ground and your left leg is stretched out behind you. Palms are flat on the floor. This is asana nine.

10. You're almost done! Asana ten is where you come back into the position and are hugging your calves. Bring your left leg up so that you're squatting. Gently raise your behind in the air until your legs are straight and your head is facing down.

11. Rise up in asana eleven and stretch back as you did in asana two.

12. Now bring your arms down in front of you slowly and put your palms together, feet hips width apart, facing forward.

Repeat this for two minutes, about two or three repetitions, and then move into other poses. You'll notice that your heart rate was elevated and you may even be perspiring a little bit. That's good! You're burning calories and you've warmed up your body for some of the more difficult exercises.

Archer Pose (★★★★☆)

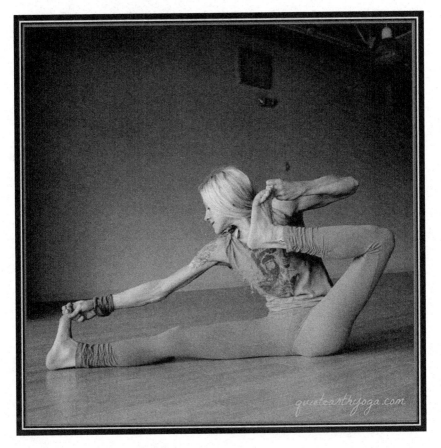

Photo courtesy of Amy at Flickr.com

The archer pose will strengthen your arms, abs, and back, and it will stretch those hamstrings as well as your calves.

1. To begin, sit in the staff position with your legs extended in front of you and your back straight. Reach forward and grab a hold of your toes and bend your

knees gently if you have to in order to keep your back from rounding.

2. Exhale and use your right hand to pull your right foot close to your torso as you bend your knee. Keep your left arm and leg in their original positions. If you feel that this is enough, stay in this position.

3. If you feel you can go further, bring your right heel closer to your right ear and extend your lifted leg out as straight as you can.

4. To come out of the pose, exhale, and release your foot and extend it back to the floor.

5. Now do the other side!

Bird of Paradise (★★★★★)

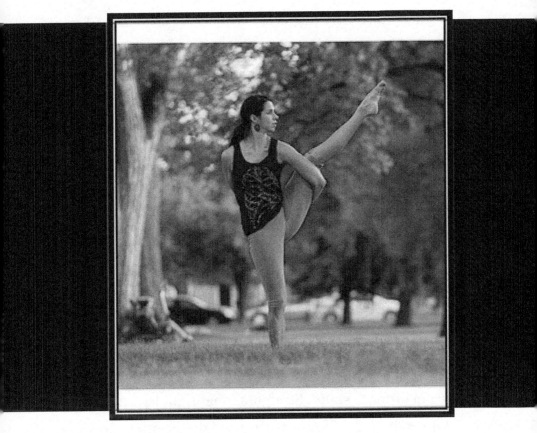

Photo courtesy of a4gpa at Flickr.com

The bird of paradise pose will strengthen your legs and stretch your inner thighs, hips, groin, shoulders and chest. It will also lengthen your spine. It's good for people who have a scattered mind, poor balance, and need more grace.

1. Begin in the mountain pose. Step your feet apart widely and turn your right leg out ninety degrees and your left leg in by forty-five degrees.

2. Raise your arms out to the sides at your shoulders and look to your right. Bend your right knee to ninety degrees and come into the virabhadrasana II pose.

3. Now, put your right hand on the floor inside your right foot with your fingertips pointed the same direction as your toes. Place your right sin and your right arm together. Reach your left arm up and extend it overhead to the right with your palm facing down.

4. Lower your left arm behind you and bend the elbow so that you can put your left palm on your right thigh. Interlace your hands behind you.

5. Now, gaze at the floor and bend your right knee and lift your right leg. Keep the knee bent. Straighten your left leg in order to stand. Straighten that right leg and hold for two breaths. Slowly release and do the other side.

Boat (★★☆☆☆)

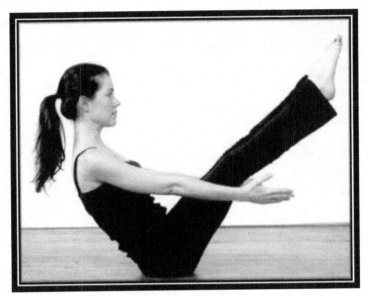

Photo courtesy of tongerandy at photobucket.com

The boat position is great to use to strengthen your abs, back and thighs. It helps with a weak core, balance, focus, self-confidence, and bloating.

1. To begin, sit on the floor and keep your knees bent but your feet flat on the floor. Grab your legs under your thighs.
2. Lean back a little and lift your feet off the floor. Keep them pressed together and lift until your shins are parallel to the floor.
3. Extend your arms straight at shoulder height with your palms facing each other.

4. Straighten your legs until you've formed a 'v' shape and balance on your glutes, not your lower back.

5. Hold this position for three to five breaths and then gently lower your shins first, and your hands on your thighs.

Bound Angle (★☆☆☆☆)

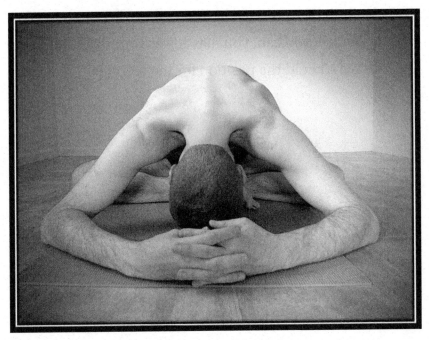

Photo courtesy of Nicholas A. Tonelli at Flickr.com

While it may not look difficult at first, you'll be surprised by how hard it is to get into this position. However, once you do, you'll realize that it's stretching your hips, thighs, groin, and lengthening your spine. This position has been known to help with anxiety, fatigue, and sciatica.

1. Come to a sitting position with your soles of your feet touching. Take hold of your big toes with your first and two fingers and thumb. Bring your heels close to your groin area.

2. Lower your knees to the floor and stretch your spine tall and straight. Now, gently bend forward until you reach the limit of your stretch. Remember, do not go too far!

3. If you feel you can, you may lower your forehead to the floor and hold the position for ten seconds.

Bow (★★★☆☆)

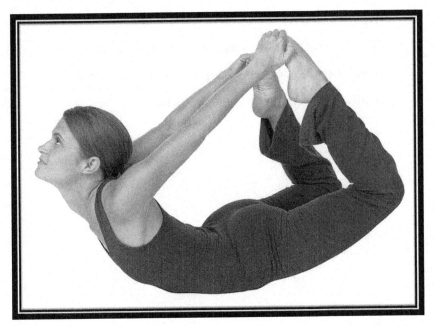

Photo courtesy of IDIA 642 Images at Flickr.com

The bow is a great move that will stretch out your entire body and strengthen your core as well as keep your spine flexible. It helps with those who are feeling fatigued.

1. Lay down on the floor front down. Lift your chest and rest your forearms parallel to each other in front of you. Come into the sphinx pose.

2. Bend your right leg and reach back to grab your right ankle with your right hand. Do the same with your left.

3. Keep your feet flexed and raise your chest off the floor and lift both of your knees. Breathe deeply and hold for five seconds.

4. To come out of the pose, gently let go of your ankles and slide your legs down. Then relax your arms and your front and lie down for a few seconds.

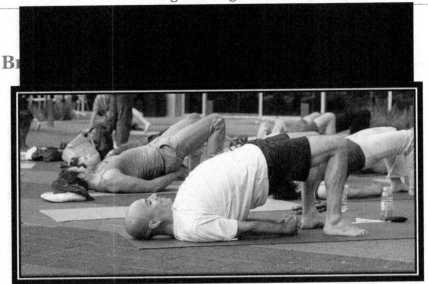

Photo courtesy of adrian Valenzuela at Flickr.com

The bridge position is excellent for your back, thighs, glutes chest, hips, quads, and your spine. It helps with intestinal function as well as anxiety and fatigue.

1. Lie down on your back and put your feet flat on the floor. Place your arms beside you with your palms down.
2. Start by lifting your torso up off the ground vertebrae by vertebrae until all of your weight is on your shoulders.
3. Now interlace your hands beneath and behind you and draw your glutes toward your knees.
4. Hold for five seconds and separate your arms slowly to slide out of the position.

Ca

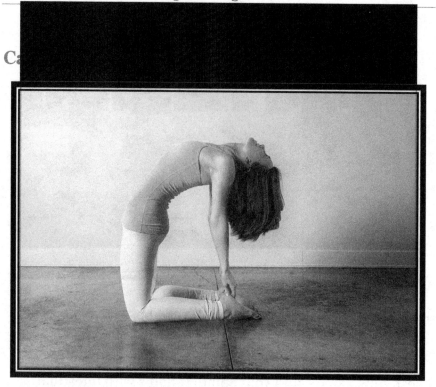

Photo courtesy of Jon Fife at Flickr.com

The camel pose may seem easy to perform, but it's a good workout for your chest, abs, groin, and thighs. This position is recommended for those who suffer from depression and poor posture.

1. Kneel on the floor with your hips directly above your knees. Your shoulders should be above your hips so you are sitting straight.

2. Place your palms on the small of your back and have your fingertips facing up. If you are not comfortable, you can put your fingertips facing the ground, too.

3. Inhale and lengthen your spine. Expand your chest and slowly lower yourself backward until you are able to grip your ankles. Try to form a square.

4. Hold this position as you breathe deeply for five seconds. To come out of the post, you can slowly slide backward until you're touching the floor and slide your legs out from under you, or you can gently pull yourself back up into a kneeling position. Whatever is comfortable for you.

Chair Pose (★★☆☆☆)

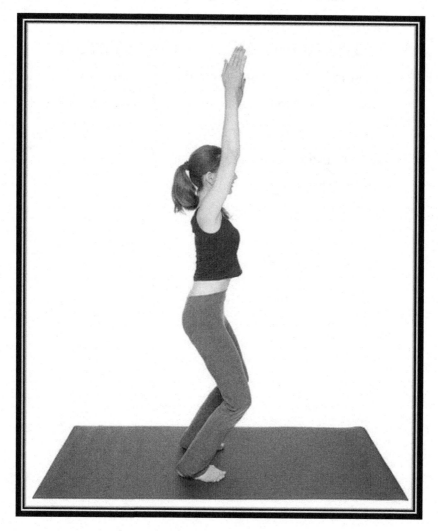

Photo courtesy of dgilder at Flickr.com

The chair pose is another deceivingly simple looking pose that is actually rather difficult considering it uses your upper back strength, glutes, thighs, calves, and ankles. This posture is excellent for posture, timidity, and endurance.

1. Get into a standing position and keep your arms at your side, or the mountain position.

2. Bend your knees deeply and shift your weight back onto your heels. Squeeze your inner thighs together.

3. Straighten your arms and raise them overhead. Bring your back into a slight bend as if you were going to sit in a chair, and hold that position.

4. Hold for ten breaths at the very least.

C

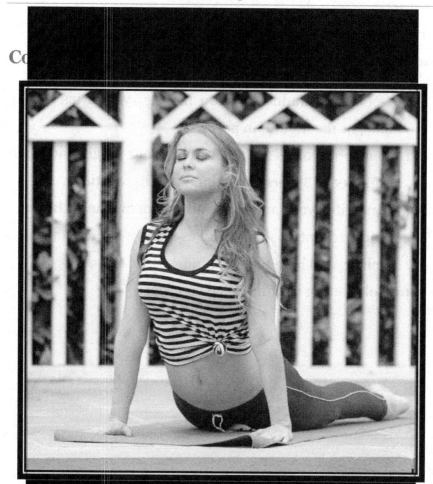

Photo courtesy of manujadon007 at photobucket.com

The full cobra position is a lot more difficult to perform because it works your thighs, glutes, hamstrings, abs, back, and your chest all at the same time. It looks pretty easy, but it's actually strenuous. This pose is excellent for those who suffer from poor posture, depression, low energy and lower back discomfort.

1. Lay down on the floor with your front on the floor. Press your toes and forehead to the floor gently. Rest your palms on either side of your chest and your finger pointing forward.

2. Lift your shoulders and chest off the floor using your palms and your arms to lift upward.

3. Keep your chest up and extend all the way up until your arms are straight. Do not allow the elbow to bend outward, keep them straight. This can cause tennis elbow if not done correctly.

4. Now make sure your hips are lifted off the ground too and your glutes are tight.

5. Breathe deeply for five breaths and gently lower back down to the ground.

Cobra Modified (★★☆☆☆)

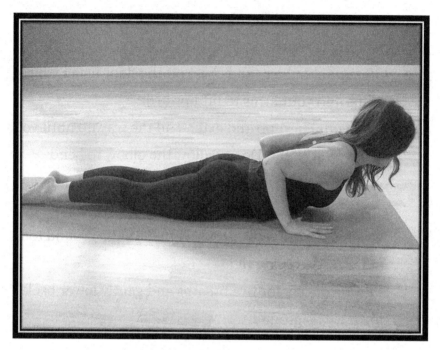

Photo courtesy of yogamama at Flickr.com

The modified cobra is a little easier to perform but still helps strengthen your back, glutes, hamstrings, chest, and abs. It's also great for posture, your back, depression, and fatigue.

1. Lay face down on the floor and press your toes and forehead to the floor.
2. Rest your palm on either side of your chest and keep your elbows bent.
3. Now press toward the floor lightly and come up until your upper arms are parallel to the floor. Bring your

palms off the floor a moment and then place them back down gently.

Cow Face (★★★★☆)

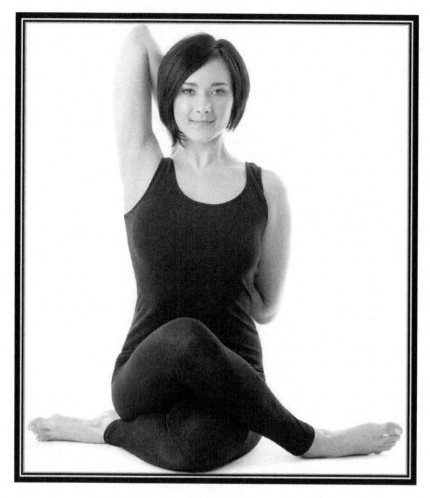

Photo courtesy of Melanie Sarta at Flickr.com

The cow face position is great for your shoulders, chest, armpits, hips, and ankles. It's for poor posture and tight shoulders.

1. Sit with your legs straight out in front of you.

2. Bend your right leg and cross it over your left. Now bend your left leg in and stack your knees with your left foot next to your right hip.

3. Now reach behind you with your left hand over your left shoulder and your right hand behind your back. Clasp your hands together and hold the position for five breaths. Switch your legs and your arms and do the other side.

4. If you want to get crazy, bend forward while doing this for an extra stretch, but only if you're comfortable with the first position!

Crescent Lunge (★★★☆☆)

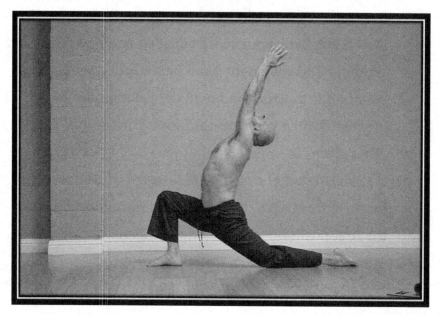

Photo courtesy of Clive Beavis at Fickr.com

The crescent lunge is excellent for your legs, hips, and balance.

1. Being in downward facing dog.

2. Step your right foot between your hands and lower your hips. Lower your left knee to the floor and untuck your toes. Press the top of your left foot into the floor.

3. Bring your arms up and overhead and touch your palms together. Bend back gently and clasp your hands. Deepen the backbend and keep your abs tight. Then return to an upright position.

4. Hold for five breaths and then gently slide out of the pose, back into downward facing dog.

Cross-Legged Forward Bend (★★★☆☆)

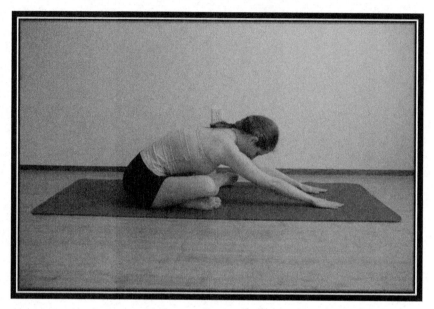

Photo courtesy of Tiffany Berry at Flickr.com

This pose is great for your hips, back shoulders, thighs, and your spine. Most people use this pose for meditation and stress.

1. Sit in a cross-legged position. Inhale and exhale deeply three times and then place your hands on the floor in front of you. Lift your hips as you do so.
2. Now bend over your legs gently as far as you can go and rest there for another three breaths, or as long as you're comfortable.
3. Sit up gently, inhaling and exhaling three times.

4. You can stay in this pose as long as you wish while you meditate.

Crow (★★★★★)

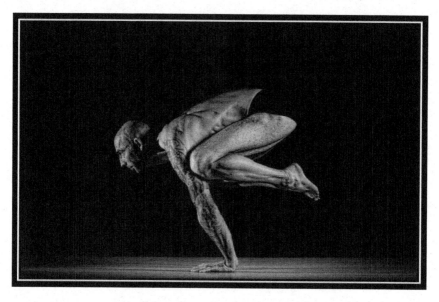

Photo courtesy of Christian Eberle at Flickr.com

Deceptively simple looking, the crow is great for strengthening your arms, shoulders, chest, abs and back. It's good to use if you suffer from a weak back, bad posture, coordination, and focus.

1. Begin in a deep squat, also known as malasana.
2. Put your hands on the floor in front of you, they should line up with your shoulders. Come up onto your tiptoes and walk your feet closer to your hands. Shift your weight forward into your hands and bring your knees up onto your elbows.

3. You may not be able to get your knees up to your elbows on the first few tries, so keep them on your elbows if you must instead.

4. Hold this position for three breaths and then gently slide out of it the way you got into it.

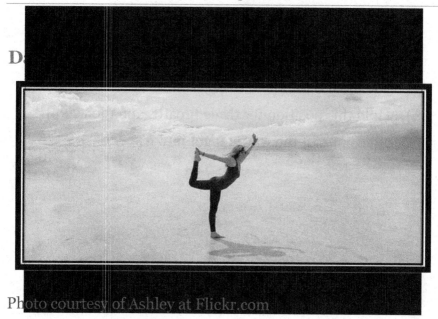

Photo courtesy of Ashley at Flickr.com

The dancer pose is most likely one of the most infamous yoga poses. It's great for your ankles, legs, thighs, groin, hips, abs, chest, shoulders and spine. People perform this pose to help with their balance, poise, energy levels, and stamina.

1. Stand in the mountain pose. Keep your feet in line with your hips and your hands by your sides.

2. Bend your right knee and reach back. Lift your right leg up and grasp your right ankle with your right hand. Try to come up as far as possible.

3. To keep your balance, reach your left hand out with your fingers pointed directly out and stay parallel with the ground.

4. Hold the position for five breaths and then switch to the other side.

Double Big Toe Hold (★★★☆☆)

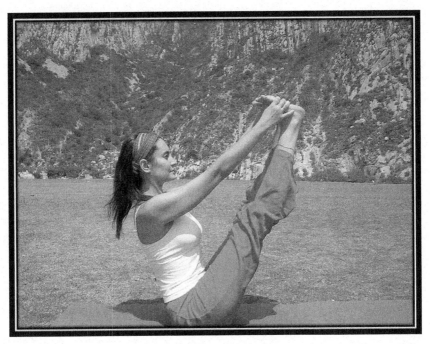

Photo courtesy of luisdemiguel at Flickr.com

The key to this position is balance. It helps with strengthening your core, legs, back, hamstrings, calves, and your spine. People use this pose to help with their balance, poise, and self-confidence.

1. Sit on the floor with your knees bent and your feet flat on the floor. Your hands should be on your knees.

2. Now, gently raise your legs in the air, keeping them parallel with one another. Grasp your big toes with both hands, using your two first fingers and your thumb to

do so. Form a 'v' shape and hold for as long as comfortable.

3. Gently let go of your toes and slide out of the position when you're finished.

Down-Dog-To-Plank Sequence (★☆☆☆☆)

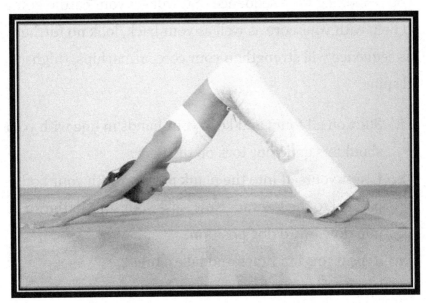

Photo courtesy of yogagirl1_bucket at photobucket.com

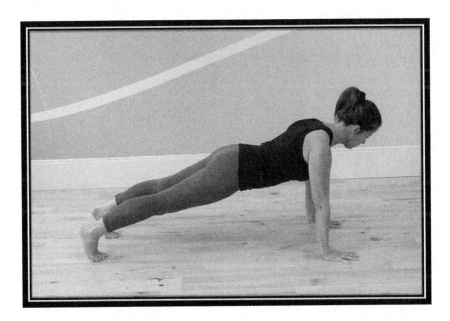

Photo courtesy of yogamama at Flickr.com

If you're looking for a sequence that will get your cardio going and help with your core as well as your back, look no further. This sequence will strengthen your core, arms, hips, thighs, and spine.

1. Start on all fours and keep your hands in line with your shoulders and your toes on the floor.
2. Lower yourself into the plank position with your body parallel to the ground. Now raise your hips in the air into downward dog position.
3. Repeat this ten times and take a break.

Eagle (★★★★★)

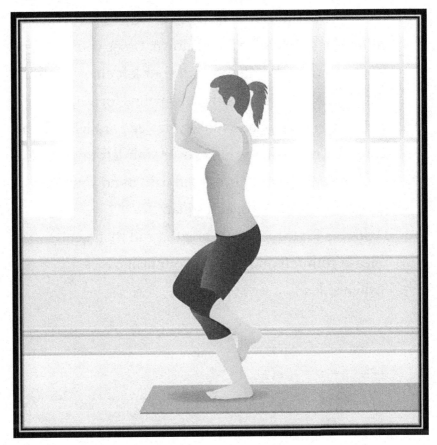

Photo courtesy of Gaurav Mishra at Flickr.com

The eagle position is great for strengthening your ankles, knees, thighs, abs, and stretching your upper back. People perform it to help with their self-confidence, as well as their poise and legs.

1. Begin in the mountain pose with your feet in line with your shoulders and your arms to your sides.

2. Raise your arms out to be parallel with the ground and your palms should be facing down. Cross your arms in front of you at the elbows with your left elbow on top. Bend your elbows and bring the palms together.

3. Lift your right foot and make your leg parallel with the ground. Cross your right leg over your left thigh and hook your toes behind your left calf. Bend your left knee, lower your hips, and squat.

4. Hold this for three to five breaths and then gently release your left and untwist your arms.

5. Switch sides.

Extended Big Toe Hold (★★★★☆)

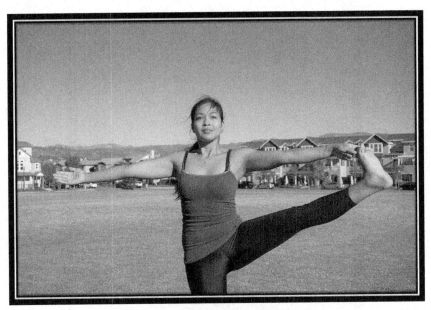

Photo courtesy of 805 Promo at Flickr.com

The extended toe hold is great for balance and poise. It stretches your legs, ankles, knees, abs, back and hamstrings.

1. Come to the mountain pose with your arms at your sides. Bring your right foot up your left leg slowly and extend your right arm so that it's parallel to the ground.
2. Extend your right leg so that it is parallel to the ground and grasp your right toe with your right hand using the first two fingers and your thumb.
3. Hold for five breaths and then release gently.
4. Switch sides.

Extended Side Angle (★★★★☆)

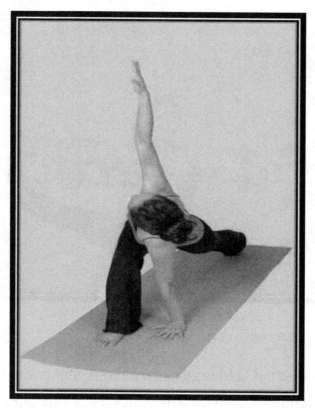

Photo courtesy of bryankestteacherstraining at photobucket.com

The extended side angle is excellent for strengthening your ankles, legs, core, upper arms, legs, hips, chest, and shoulders. People perform the pose for endurance, breathing, focus, their sciatica, and digestion.

1. Begin by standing in warrior pose II, found <u>here</u>.

2. Lower your left hand to the floor inside of your left foot and reach your right arm up.

3. Rotate your right arm by using our shoulder blade and extend your body into one long line from the outside of your right foot through the fingertips of your right hand, as shown.

4. Hold for five breaths and then gently twist your core so that you're straight and slide your leg back to be parallel with the ground.

5. Switch sides.

Firefly (★★★★★)

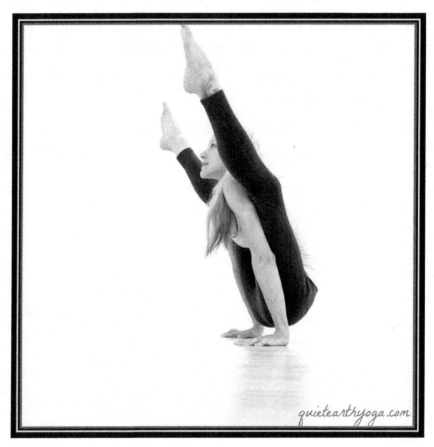

Photo courtesy of Amy at Flickr.com

The firefly pose is excellent for strengthening your arms, shoulders, abs, wrists, and hamstrings.

1. Start in a wide-legged squat and your hands in front of you on the floor.

2. Wrap your hands behind and around your feet and reach your shoulders under your knees.

3. Lift your feet and put your weight onto your hands.

4. Hold for three breaths and gently slide your legs out of the position, slowly.

Fish (★★☆☆☆)

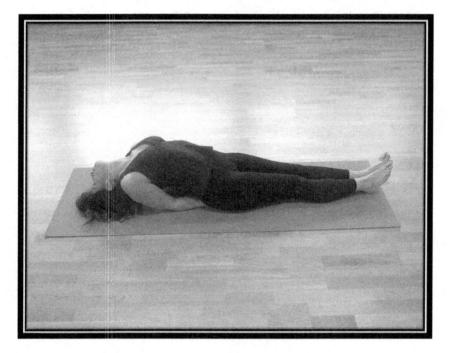

Photo courtesy of yogamama at Flickr.com

Another deceptively easy looking yoga position, but should only be performed by intermediate level yogis. The fish position is great for your chest, neck, hips, and upper back.

1. Lie on the floor on your back and keep your toes pointed skyward. Your arms should be alongside your body.

2. Now, place your palms on the floor and press your elbows into the floor. Arch your upper back and try to reach your heart toward the ceiling.

3. Pull your shoulders blade together and lift your chin.

4. Lean to the left and bring our right arm under your glutes and to the same for the other side. Hold for five breaths and gently slide out of the position.

Forearm Balance (★★★★☆)

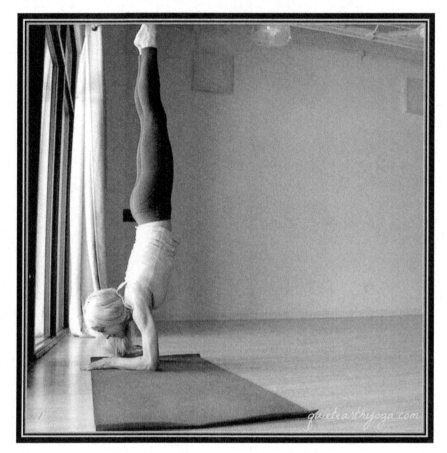

Photo courtesy of Amy at Flickr.com

The forearm balance is excellent for strengthening your core, arms, shoulders, back and chest. People use this for anxiety, fear, bad habits, and change of perspective.

1. Kneel with your behind resting on your heels. Place your forearms on the floor in front of you and keep them shoulder width apart.

2. Straighten your legs into dolphin pose.

3. Now lift your left foot toward the ceiling and lift your right leg up next. Squeeze your legs together and point your toes. Hold for two breaths and gently slide out of the position.

Frog (★★★☆☆)

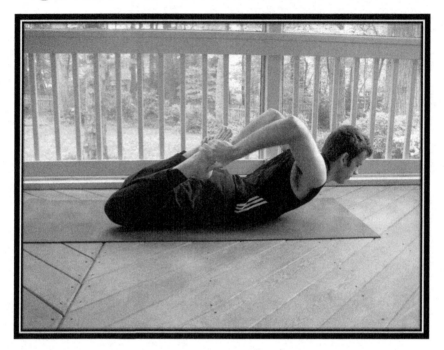

Photo courtesy of Chris at Flickr.com

The frog position strongly resembles the bow position and is also great for your thighs, hips and groin. People use this for digestion problems and knee pain.

1. Begin by getting on all fours and keep your knees at a wide stance. Lean forward as you lower your core to the floor.
2. Now rest your forearms on the floor and keep your torso above the floor.

3. Lower your torso until your body is on the floor and reach back to grasp your ankles.

4. Hold the position for four breaths and then release.

Half Moon (★☆☆☆☆)

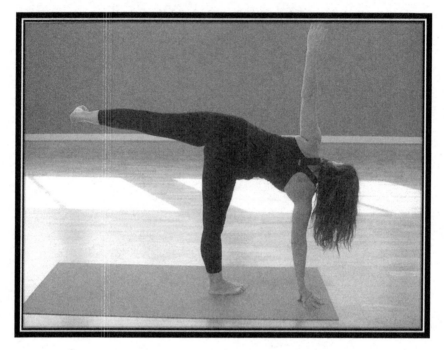

Photo courtesy of yogamama at Flickr.com

The half-moon position is great for your back, abs, knees, buttocks and hips. Yogis use it for balance endurance, self-confidence, and a scattered mind.

1. Begin in the triangle pose and keep your right leg in front.
2. Lower your left hand to your hip and put your right fingertips on the floor.
3. Lift your right leg into the air and straighten it.

4. Lift your right arm into the air and reach toward the sky.

5. Hold the position for five breaths and switch sides.

Handstand (★★★★☆)

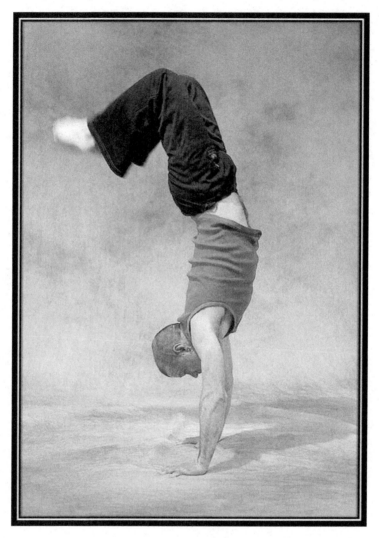

Photo courtesy of Patty Townsend at Flickr.com

A move that requires discipline and amazing balance, the handstand is not one that you want to try pulling off when you're a beginner. You can easily overcompensate and topple.

This move is excellent for your shoulders, arms, wrists, core, legs, abs, and spine.

1. Place your hands on the floor in front of you and come into a downward facing dog pose.
2. Now do a few hops with each foot to get into position. When you're ready, hop up so that your feet are pointing to the ceiling, your head is hanging between your arms, and your arms are straight.
3. Hold the position for ten seconds and then release. You can rotate your hips if you're comfortable.

Happy Baby (★★☆☆☆)

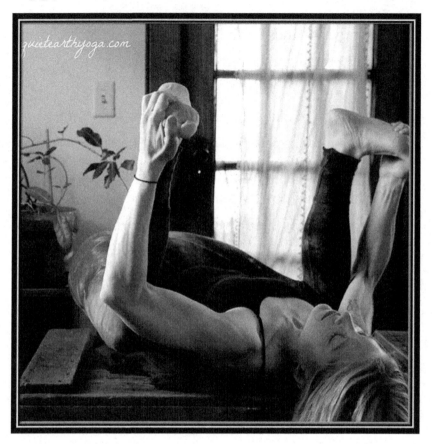

Photo courtesy of Amy at Flickr.com

The happy baby position is great for your inner thighs, groin, knees, and lower back. It helps with lower back discomfort and tight hips.

1. Lie down on your back and bring your knees up into a bent position. Keep your feet flat on the floor and your palms should be facing up.

2. Now bend your knees to your chest and separate them to the sides. Hold your shins or your toes with your fingers and bring your thighs down until they're parallel with the floor.

3. You should be able to bring your thighs down next to your torso, but don't stretch too far if you're not comfortable.

4. Hold for five breaths and then release.

Headstand (★★★★★)

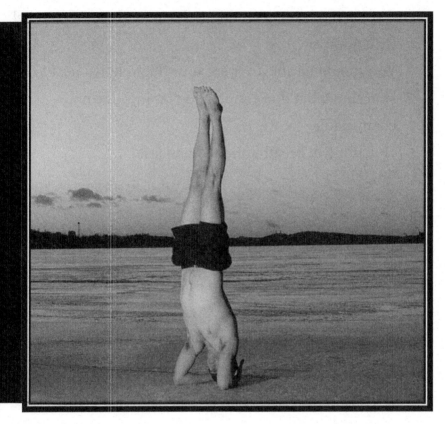

Photo courtesy of Sami Taipale at Flickr.com

The headstand requires a little less balance than the handstand, but it's still pretty difficult to perform when you're an adult. This is also great for your core, legs, spine, and arms.

1. Start with downward facing dog.

2. Move into dolphin pose and lower your forearms to the floor. Interlace your fingers together so that your arms form a triangle.

3. Now gently raise your legs above you, this may take a few tries, and hold for ten seconds. Keep your core tight and your legs tight.

4. Slide out of the pose gently and be careful not to fall.

Locust (★★★★☆)

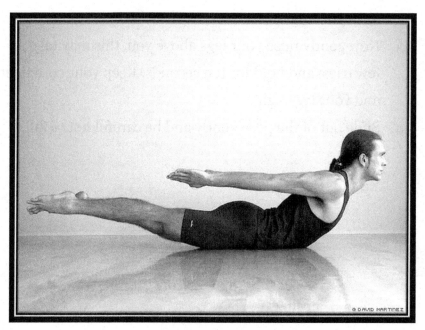

Photo courtesy of On Being at Flickr.com

It looks easy and pretty streamlined, but the locust pose is hard on your core and thigh muscles. It strengthens your back, buttocks, chest, shoulders, spine and helps with back pain as well as posture.

1. Lie face down on the floor and keep your arms alongside you with your palms facing up.
2. Bring your chest off the floor and keep your chin parallel to the ground.

3. Raise your arms to your chest and keep them parallel to the ground. Now raise your legs off the floor and keep your feet together.

4. Inhale and exhale a few times with your core muscles tightened and your buttocks tense.

5. Then slowly release.

Locust Variation (★★★★☆)

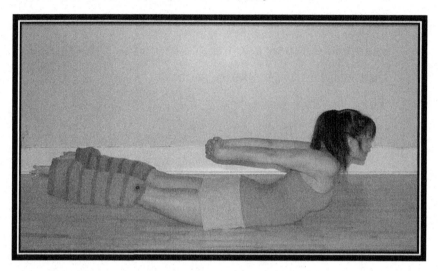

Photo courtesy of Elsie Escobar at Flickr.com

If you're comfortable with the first variation of the locust pose, try this one.

1. Come into the locust pose mentioned earlier, but place your arms behind your back and interlace your fingers together. This will stretch your shoulder blades and your chest.

Monkey (★★★★★)

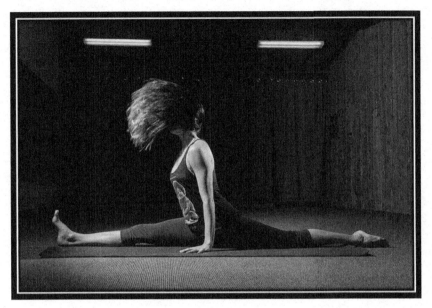

Photo courtesy of a4gpa at Flickr.com

The monkey pose looks easy until you try to get your groin to touch the floor. This pose will strengthen your legs, hips, and help with your sciatica.

1. Start by getting on all fours and step your right foot between your hands.
2. Stretch your left leg out behind you and place the top of your foot onto the floor.
3. Stretch your right leg out in front of you and place the back of your heel on the floor. Keep your arms straight beside you and rest your palms on the floor.

4. Your torso should be straight and your groin should be touching the floor, but go only as far as is comfortable.

5. Hold for five breaths and gently draw your outward-facing leg in, and your inward facing leg in next.

6. Switch sides.

One-Legged King Pigeon (★★★★★)

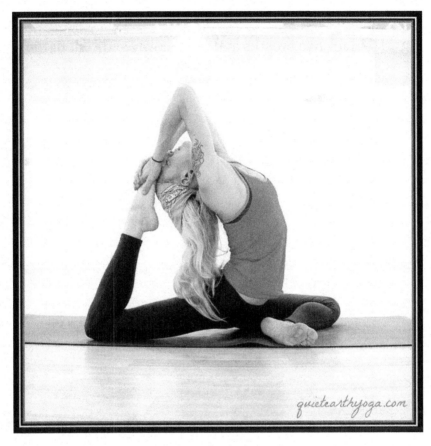

Photo courtesy of Amy at Flickr.com

The one-legged king pigeon looks difficult to perform, but it's still not considered advanced. This is helpful for your thighs, hips, groin, neck, shoulders and spine. If you have a thyroid condition, consider using this pose.

1. Start with the pigeon pose, found <u>here</u>.

2. Sit up tall, firm your abs, and scissor your thighs. Bend your left knee and grab your left foot with your left hand. Bring it up to the back of your head gently.

3. Hold for five breaths and then slowly slide out of the pose.

4. Switch Sides.

Peacock (★★★★☆)

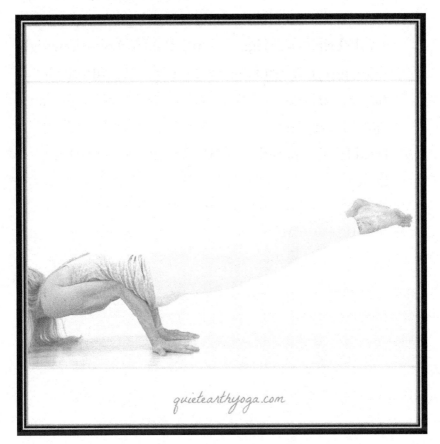

quietearthyoga.com

Photo courtesy of Amy at Flickr.com

The peacock pose will help you strengthen your core, upper body, shoulders, and neck. It's great for relieving stress, depression, and anxiety.

1. Start on all fours and place your hands directly under your shoulders. Your fingertips should be pointing toward you.

2. Straighten your legs behind you and get into the plank position.

3. Now bend your elbows at a ninety-degree angle and gently bring your right leg into the air. Lower our right side onto your right elbow. Do the same with the left side. Keep your legs together and in the air, pointing out behind you.

4. Hold for five breaths and then gently lower to the ground.

Pendant Pose (★★★★☆)

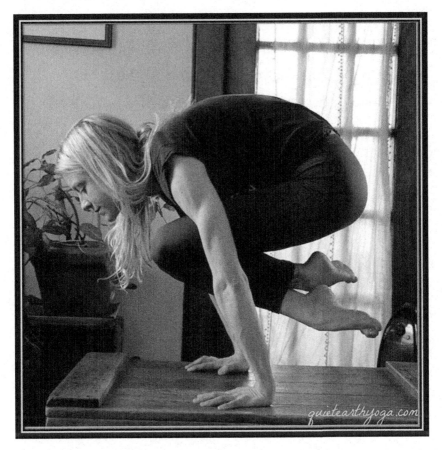

Photo courtesy of Amy at Flickr.com

The pendant pose is an excellent addition to anyone's routine as long as they're able to balance well. It's beneficial for the back, upper body strength, and abs.

1. Start in the cow face pose with your legs crossed and your right knee over your lef.t

2. Then place your palms on the floor at your shoulders and lift your hips off your heels by leaning into your palms.

3. Now look down, lift your hips higher and press firmly into the palms as you lift the feet off the floor.

4. Hold for two or three breaths and then lower back down. Switch sides with your legs and repeat.

Plank (★★☆☆☆)

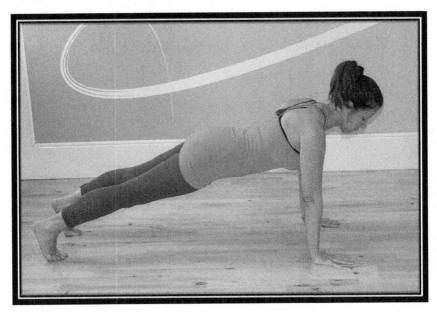

Photo courtesy of yogamama at Flickr.com

The plank is excellent for strengthening your core and your upper arms, as well as lengthening your spine. The pose focuses on helping you strengthen, posture, breathing, and endurance.

1. Begin on all fours with your palms at shoulder width and your knees in line with your hips.
2. Now press into your palms and straighten your legs out behind you, starting with your right and ending with your left. Keep your arms straight and your legs straight.

3. Use your core to keep from moving and hold for five breaths. Gently lower yourself to the ground and rest for two breaths.

4. Come back up into the plank position again, repeat this process three times.

Plow (★★★★☆)

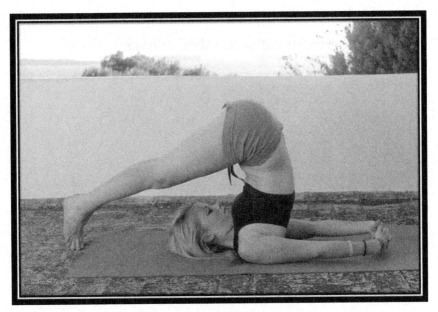

Photo courtesy of yogamama at Flickr.com

The plow will help you stretch your back, neck, hamstrings, shoulders and keep your spine flexible. It's also good for hormonal balance, your thyroid, and insomnia.

1. Lie on your back and keep your knees bent and your feet flat on the floor. Stretch your arms out alongside your body with your palms pressing into the floor.
2. Bring your knees toward your chest and extend your legs over your head. Touch the balls of your feet to the floor behind you.
3. Clasp your hands behind you.

4. Bend your knees and place your right knee next to your right ear and your left knee next to your left ear. Release your hands and bring them up to rest next to your feet. Hold for five breaths and then release.

Rabbit (★★★★☆)

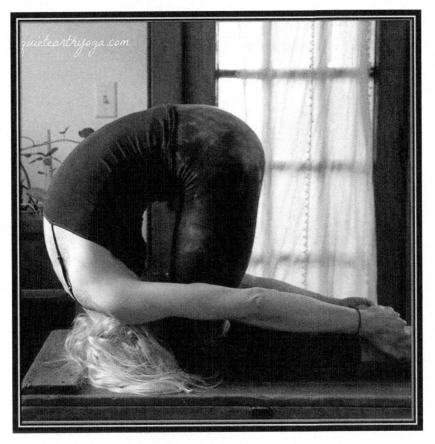

Photo courtesy of Amy at Flickr.com

The rabbit pose will help you stretch your entire body and lengthen your spine. It's also used for headaches, spinal tension, insomnia, neck pain, back pain, and digestion.

1. Start in child's pose and grab the outside edges of your ankles. Roll from your forehead to the crown of your head and inhale and exhale slowly.

2. Extend your arms and shift your body weight forward and onto your head.

3. Reach your arms back so that you're grasping your ankles still and hold this pose for three breaths.

4. Release and relax before you go into the next pose.

Reclining Hero (★☆☆☆☆)

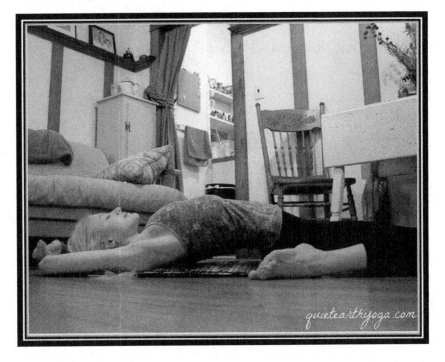

Photo courtesy of Amy at Flickr.com

The reclining hero looks very relaxing, and it is if you're not a beginner. If you're not flexible at this point, do not attempt this pose as it may harm your upper thigh muscles. The reclining hero is used for stretching the tops of your feet, quads, ankles, and abs. It's to help with low energy and fatigue, menstrual pain, and leg flexibility.

1. Start by kneeling on the floor and separating your feet behind you. Lower your butt to the floor between your legs and then slowly slide back.

2. Rest your shoulder blades on the floor behind you and your arms at yours sides with your palms facing up.

3. Breathe deeply for as long as you'd like and then slide your legs forward when you're finished.

Reverse Plank (★★★☆☆)

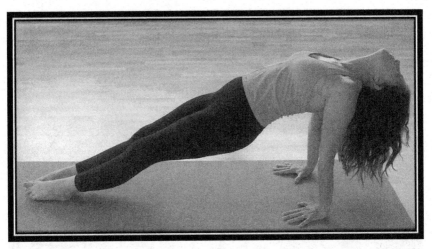

Photo courtesy of yoga mama at Flickr.com

The reverse plank is to strengthen your arms, legs, wrists, and ankles. It also stretches your abs, chest, shoulders, and thighs.

1. Sit straight with your legs out in front of you and your heels touching.
2. Place your hands on the floor in line with your shoulders and your palms facing down. Your fingers should be pointed toward your toes. Now lift your hips until your entire body is straight and your heels are touching the floor.
3. If it's more comfortable, let your head drop back and hold this position for ten deep breaths.
4. Release and repeat five times.

Reverse Warrior (★★★☆☆)

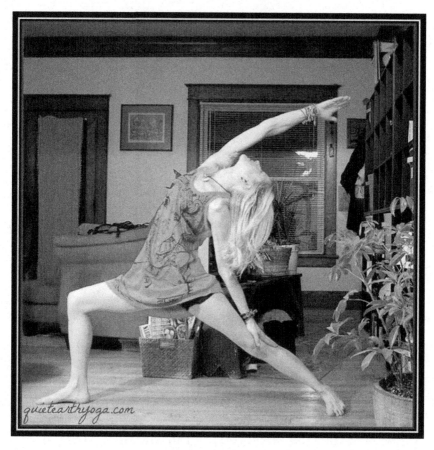

Photo courtesy of Amy at Flickr.com

The reverse warrior looks simple, but having good balance is key here. This is to strengthen your abs, thighs, hips, groin, and keep your spine flexible. Yogis use this pose to ease lower back pain and fatigue.

1. Start in the warrior II pose found <u>here</u>.

2. Now lower your left hand back to your left leg and slide it toward your ankle. Go as far as possible and turn your body to the ceiling. Arch your right arm overhead.

3. This may be as far as you can go, but if you feel comfortable, try to go further.

4. Turn your gaze up and lower your right arm and lift your left arm until they're both at shoulder height.

5. Return to Warrior II pose and then switch sides.

Shoulder Stand (★★★★☆)

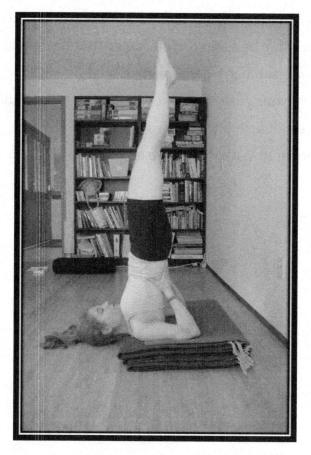

Photo courtesy of Tiffany Berry at Flickr.com

The key to this pose is to stay straight as you're doing it, which is harder than it looks. The pose is excellent for strengthening your upper back, abs, neck, shoulders and arms. It stretches your back and shoulders and helps your circulatory system as well as your thyroid.

1. Lie with your arms at your sides with the palms facing up. You should be on your back. Your feet should be shoulder width apart.

2. While keeping your feet together, raise them off the floor and use your hands on your lower back to support you.

3. Straighten your spine and legs. Breathe deeply and hold the pose for five breaths before sliding out of it like you got into it.

Reference Poses

Warrior Pose II (★☆☆☆☆)

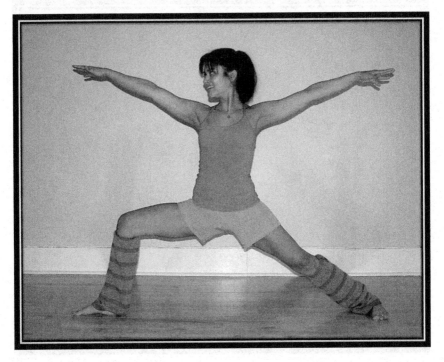

Photo courtesy of Elsie Escobar at Flickr.com

Pigeon Pose (★★★☆☆)

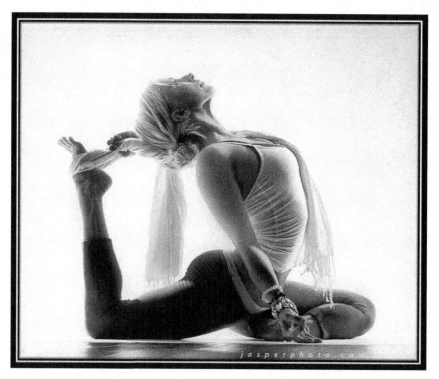

Photo courtesy of Kukhahn Yoga at Flickr.com

Conclusion

Yoga is excellent for your body and your overall health. It helps to lower your stress levels and become in touch with your body and how it's performing. Many people report that after performing yoga for a few weeks, their muscles no longer ache and they're able to sleep better at night. So if you're someone who suffers from muscles and joint aches, insomnia, headaches, abdominal upset, and any other physical or mental ailment, yoga will be good for you.

Remember that while some of these poses look easy to perform, they will put strain on your muscles and your back, so be sure that you've warmed up and you're stretched before you begin. Hydration is also a big part of staying safe and fluid while you're performing yoga, so don't forget to bring a water of bottle.

If you liked this eBook on Yoga Poses, ***please leave a positive review here***. It will only take 1 minute but it is extremely important to me.

Thank you for reading!

With love and respect,

Roberto Zanon

CPSIA information can be obtained
at www.ICGtesting.com
Printed in the USA
FSOW04n2158050116
15458FS